The Mindful Walker

The *Mindful* Walker

REDISCOVERING THE SIMPLE PATH TO A HEALTHIER, HAPPIER, MORE PEACEFUL LIFE

Alex Strauss

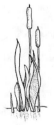

"In every walk with nature, one receives far more than he seeks."—John Muir

Contents

Thanks!

To Thank you for choosing my book, I invite you to take advantage of these FREE additional resources to support you on your journey toward a more mindful experience of the Natural world:

- A 10-Minute mp3 guided mindful walk

- A printable walking journal and walking log

- Direct links to some of my best video trainings

- References for the scientific studies mentioned in this book

- Other things I may have added since I wrote this edition!

Access them all at
TheMindfulWalker.com/BookBonuses

For Gretchen, Annika, & Dave
Thanks for always encouraging me to walk . . .
even when it meant you had to clean up
the supper dishes.

Foreword

It is time to bring our awareness back to the Natural World.

First, experiencing nature connectedness will make us happier, healthier and more at peace —science has proven it.

Second, practicing mindfulness will make us wiser, better informed, and more compassionate. And third, when we connect, we care. People protect what they love, and a true love of Nature will inspire solutions to the creation of a more sustainable world.

Alex Strauss has combined her love of walking mindfully in Nature with her passion for empowering people. Don't be fooled by the simplicity, though. The path Alex invites us to follow points to something profound and beautiful. The words on the page invite you to get up, get out and follow in her footsteps on your own journey. They point to something truly special —a chance to gain a new perspective on the world around us and a greater understanding of our role in it.

To Alex, thank you for sharing your unique connection and natural wisdom. To you reading my words, enjoy your journey with Nature and *The Mindful Walker.*

— Ian Banyard, Author, *Natural Mindfulness: Your Personal Guide to the Healing Power of Nature Connection*

April 2020

Introduction

When I published the first edition of *The Mindful Walker* in 2016, I was flying high.

As the fog of my months-long depression lifted and my energy soared, I was walking on sunshine. I felt as though I had discovered the "keys to the kingdom" in my daily mindful walks and I couldn't wait to tell everyone about it. I talked about it. I made audio meditations. I set up a YouTube channel and a website. (None of which I knew how to do.) I wrote like the wind about my newfound discovery of the miraculous healing power of Nature.

To my disappointment, not everyone wanted to hear it. Either they already felt "guilty" about the time they weren't spending outside, they didn't especially like being in Nature, or they were simply too busy and distracted to listen. Some considered my message frivolous (as if something so simple could not also be profound). Honestly, I myself, for all my enthusiasm, secretly worried that it *was* a bit frivolous. At the end of the day, we're only talking about walking mindfully in the outdoors, after all. (For a while, I took pains *not* to share it with the healthcare professionals who read the medical magazine I publish.) Some people just thought I was misguided to be making "such a big deal" about something that was... well... kind of simple and obvious.

While most reviewers loved the book (thank you, dear ones) and gave it kind reviews, there were a few who wrote things like "Duh. Go outside. Walk. You'll feel better. Nothing new here." Um. Yeah. That is actually the point.

At first, those reviews stung. I mean, I *had* devoted the better part of a year to developing the material that went into this book and I was poised to devote the rest of my professional life to preaching the benefits of mindful connection with Nature. Was I wasting my time?

But as receptivity to my message grew—and as I grew in my own understanding and practice—I started to realize how many people around the world were simultaneously waking up to these same concepts (simple and obvious, though they may be).

Interest in natural mindfulness, walking meditation, forest bathing, nature therapy, and Earth-based spirituality was and is growing rapidly. It's as though we got the same message at the same time. (Sidenote: This *does* actually happen. See *Big Magic* by Elizabeth Gilbert)

People from all walks of life are stepping out of their homes and offices and into natural spaces at record rates. We are being drawn back to the Earth by a desire to repair both it and ourselves. Fortunately, for those of us with some serious right-brain tendencies, the science backs up what instinct seems to be telling us. It turns out, we actually *need* to connect with the more-than-human world for optimal physical, psychological, and spiritual well-being. Go figure.

As I write this, we are in the midst of a global pandemic. While humanity struggles with the implications of "social distancing", the air is quietly clearing over major cities and many are finding solace in Nature, some for the first time. Gardens are being planted, parks are being visited, and yes, many mindful walks are being taken. And even more people are feeling the effects for themselves.

Is it simple? Yes, absolutely. Is it obvious? Maybe. But don't we all need a little extra encouragement and support sometimes to do the simple, obvious things that could make our lives so much better?

I know I do.

This is a book about how to settle your busy mind and reconnect with the best part of who you are—your higher self, if you will—by walking in Nature. That's it. I'm not pretending that it is more than that. And yet, I cannot pretend that it is anything less than life-changing, if you allow it to be. The ancient practice of mindful walking transformed my own life, as it has the lives of thousands of others before me.

It took me years to understand, but here is what I now know: That feeling of "peace" we have when we walk in a forest or watch a sunset over the ocean is not something we have to save for vacation. It is not even something we have to save for our walks. The heavy sigh, the letting go, the "settling in" to ourselves. That is, in fact, the feeling of our "default setting" as human beings. We were all born with the capacity to live calm, centered lives, gently riding the ups and downs and managing problems with creativity and grace. If we can just get out of our own way.

So many of us have gradually become subtly "uprooted" by distractions and the minutiae of daily life. We are out of sync with our peaceful default setting. Ironically, while technology allows us to be *more* connected to global events and each other's day-to-day news, most of us are disconnected from our cyclical nature, the messages of our bodies, the healing power of the Earth, the impact of seasons on our psyche, and our intuitive guidance system.

But reconnection is possible, no matter how far gone you think you are. It really is possible to live in a state of more-or-less perpetual calm, enjoy a pretty constant energy level, and be able to count on your mind to cut through clutter and deliver creative ideas and wise solutions, even in the most difficult situations, so that you can feel satisfied and even joyful.

The key is to find, in the midst of the clamour of life, a way to clear our minds and reconnect with that "higher self" on a regular basis. Preferably, a way that does not require a lot of time or energy we don't have, a way that feels natural, a way that doesn't take long to master, and that won't leave us feeling exhausted. It would be a bonus if that method was also free.

Meditation can work. Yoga can work. Heck, even mindful gardening can work. You have to find what works for you. And by "works", I mean what will fit into your life as it is *right now*. Thankfully, the simple practice of moving through a natural setting in a state of present-moment awareness has the power to bring us back to ourselves, foster mental clarity, mitigate some of the negative effects of stress, spark creativity, and boost our energy. It's easy. It's free. And almost anyone can do it.

Imagine rising above the most stressful situations, tackling daily tasks with renewed energy, making easier decisions, sleeping like a baby, and waking up in a better mood. All while toning your derriere and strengthening your core. That's mindful walking. What's not to love?

Guarantee (How many books give you that?!)

If you follow the steps in this book and are willing to devote just ten minutes a few times a week to quietly walking in Nature in the way that I'll show you (no crunches, chants, or celery-based diets involved), I promise that you will cut your perceived stress level in half (or more) in the next 30 days, dramatically raise your capacity for hope and wonder, increase your focus and energy, and begin to restore that elusive feeling of contentment that is your birthright. You may even come away with a tighter rear end and more shapely calves.

It really *is* all that. Get your walking shoes ready!

1

Talking to Trees

When I was a little girl, I talked to trees.

When I thought no one was looking, I would whisper my "secrets" into their knobby trunks and fervently watch for some sign of recognition or acknowledgement. A twitch of a branch or a falling leaf was an "answer". I kissed my favorite trees and stroked their bark. I engaged in lengthy "conversations". I think I knew, even then, that some adults might find this worrisome, so I tried to keep the habit to myself. But I continued to engage in these private one-way dialogues well into my college years.

Eventually, of course, I grew out of the fantasy. I moved to the city, got a Master's degree, became a journalist, and pretty much relegated trees—and the rest of the Natural World, for that matter—to the beautiful backdrop they are for so many of us. Indoor life became "real life". Outdoors was for weekends, vacations, and an occasional jog or bike ride.

It wasn't until years later, in the midst of some significant challenges in my adult life, that I recalled those early conversations and was drawn, once again, to commune with trees. As I reacquainted myself with these old friends and felt the familiar rapport, it dawned on me that the true miracle of this relationship—a miracle that I could not have fathomed as a child—was not that I could talk to trees, but that *trees could talk to me.*

Although this book is about the many benefits of walking, it is also a book about the ways in which trees, and the rest of the more-than-human world, can communicate with us when we put ourselves in a position—literally and figuratively—to hear them. Their messages are vital for our busy lives and our troubled times. They are messages of peace, hope, strength, resilience, groundedness and *connection* not only to our world and the Universal intelligence behind it, but also to all living things and to our best selves.

Maybe you have thought, as I once did, that there is something not quite right about trying to feel peaceful and content when there is still so much wrong with the world or even in your own life. What right have we to feel good when so many are suffering? Looking back, I know there have been times when I kept myself miserable, just to prove (to whom, I'm not sure) that I *cared*.

But the truth is that acceptance of what *is* is the first vital step toward change. You don't have to like it but you do have to make peace with it before you can address it. As writer and Franciscan monk Richard Rohr writes, "Foundational love gives us hope and allows us to trust 'what is' as the jumping-off point, no matter how unsteady it feels. It allows us to work together toward 'what can be.'"

Why am I talking about this in a book about walking? Because by naturally calming the nervous system and quieting the mind, walking mindfully in Nature can put us in touch with that "foundational love"—whether you call it God, Spirit, Universe or Higher Self. It can help us not only feel more peaceful in the moment but more accepting of life in general, even while we are getting in our daily dose of physical activity. In that sense, regular exposure to Nature through walking is a smart place to start, whether your goal is to change your life, change your body, or change the world!

When I first started taking regular walks, there were a lot of things out of joint in my life. I wasn't especially healthy or happy. I was working too hard and enjoying too little. But slowing down enough to see the beauty in individual moments on my daily walks opened the space in my head for fresh insights. These insights led to many positive changes (including the writing of this book and the start of my coaching business). The trees themselves may not have given me these insights, per se, but their presence certainly did (as you'll see when we get into the science in later chapters).

So if you have been striving and trying and overthinking like mad in an effort to improve your life, get healthier, get happier, or solve some other problem, and you feel like you have been getting nowhere, I invite you to ask yourself this:

What if a less stressful, more fulfilling, and creative life requires a lot less effort than we think? What if Nature, in her wisdom, knows something we don't know about going with the flow of life? What if our lives were designed to be easier, more fun, and more joyful, but all of our striving and effort to "figure everything out" is just getting in the way? Could it be that we need to get quiet and listen to the Earth in order to hear our heart's wisdom?

I'm not sure what drew you to pick up this book. Maybe it was the promise of "peace" for busy people. Maybe it was that word "mindful" that has become such a buzzword in recent years. Perhaps you were just looking for a gentler way to exercise or lose a few pounds. Or maybe you are recovering from—or trying to ward off—an illness.

Regardless of why you're here, I want you to know that that instinct to walk in Nature is a good one. I do not believe it is accidental that you found this little book. Whatever it is you are grappling with, if you invest the hour-and-a-half or so it takes to read *The Mindful Walker*, and you implement its strategies with an open mind, the trees will surely speak to you, too.

2

Stumbling Into Wellbeing

Before I started walking in my suburban neighborhood around 2007, I had never been a "walker". As is the case for so many people, it was stress that drove me to change. My family and I had just made a big move across the country—one that had been anticipated, planned, and looked forward to. But I was in a slump. By day, I was trying to set up our new household, meet my neighbors, keep up my work as a writer and magazine editor, and run around after my two grade school-aged daughters.

By night, I just worried. I would lie in bed calculating the bills and running through a laundry list of personal or professional "problems". I worried about my kids, my bank account, my wrinkles, my business, the melting polar ice caps, poverty, you name it. Without the balancing effect of friends, routines, and the gym I was used to, worry became my constant companion. My health suffered, too. I lost weight. I was easily irritated. And very few things felt fun.

In the past, I had always taken these kinds of problems to a higher power. I was active in a church and regularly spent time in prayer. But in the early months in this unfamiliar town, my faith did not seem to be helping me much. God suddenly seemed unusually distant.

At first, I tried to tackle this intellectually. I immersed myself in learning, reading books and blogs on psychology, philosophy, spirituality, healthy habits, and simple living. Maybe I just needed to streamline my work, take up yoga again, try Buddhism, eat better, or get a new hobby. . . ? After supper, while the kids did their homework, I walked our new puppy around our wooded neighborhood, deep in thought. I was determined to figure things out if it killed me.

I walked and thought and thought and walked until my head hurt and I couldn't think anymore.

And then I just walked.

At the time, of course, I had no idea that the walking itself—such a simple, straightforward thing we all do naturally—was going to completely transform the way I approach problems, manage stress, make decisions, relate to other people, Creation, and God, and even understand myself.

But sometime during the first 100 miles or so of the 6,500 miles worth of mindful walks I have now taken, I started to see that this thing I was doing—taking short, quiet walks in a green space—was actually a powerful practice for personal wellbeing. Beyond philosophy or psychology or even religion. Seeing that changed everything.

I knew people who walked for exercise or enjoyment and those who took walks with friends to socialize. But I did not personally know anyone who intentionally practiced this particular brand of meditative movement in Nature. (For half a second I swear I thought I had *invented* mindful walking. As if.) Without changing anything else in my life and with minimal effort, I was experiencing all kinds of physical and psychological benefits.

Like any new convert, I decided that everyone should know about it. So I drew upon my broadcast background and put together a short audio program on mindful walking (which is still available for download). In the 10-minute program, I shared some of the visualizations and meditative techniques that were melting my own stress and helping me feel much more peaceful, not just while I was walking, but for hours or even days afterward.

I shared the audio program and a short ebook about

mindful walking (by this time I had discovered that this was, in fact, an ancient and time-honored practice) with friends, neighbors, people at my church, folks in my social network, and anyone else who would listen.

To my surprise and delight, they ate it up! It quickly became clear that I wasn't the only one hungry for a simple, practical way to slow down and be more mindful in the midst of a busy life. As I started to tentatively speak on the topic of mindful walking, I met a lot of people who loved the idea of a practice that could nurture their spirits, strengthen their bodies, and soothe their minds without breaking the bank or throwing a wrench into their schedules.

Some of these people were already hikers or walkers who had experienced the peace of Nature for themselves, but had never thought of making mindful walking part of their daily lives. Many were people who were looking to simplify their lives, be better stewards of the Earth, clean up their diets, manage stress better, or just get outside more. Like me at the start of my own journey, they tended to be Nature-loving seekers who felt that something was a little "off" in their lives and were anxious to find a fix. Whatever their personal motivations, these people all recognized the life-changing potential in the practice of walking mindfully in the outdoors. If you can see yourself in any of these scenarios (or even if you'd like to), I hope that you will, too!

Note: *If you would like to get a copy of the audio program I mentioned, I have included it as part of your free Book Bonuses. You'll find them all waiting for you at TheMindfulWalker.com/BookBonuses.*

CHAPTER

3

The Path of Least Resistance

At its core, mindful walking is just a more thoughtful and intentional way of approaching the simple but largely lost art of "taking a walk".

In contrast to mindless wandering—which certainly has merits of its own—mindful walking is a more disciplined practice that allows the walker to take advantage of the synergy between Movement, Mindfulness (present moment awareness), and Nature.

Like any practice, the more you engage in it, the better and more consistent your results will be.

Why Walking?

I'm not here to convince you that you'll feel happier and calmer if you are more mindful and get more fresh air and exercise. If you've picked up this book, I'm assuming you probably know that. You are likely also aware of at least some of the benefits of mindfulness and regular exercise. (We'll get to the role Nature plays in a little bit.)

Obviously, there are plenty of ways to get more of both of these things. One of the most popular routes to mindfulness is through meditation, a mental training technique which invites you to quiet the mind and release negative thoughts. Meditation practitioners often sit with eyes closed and practice turning their focus inward. Following the flow of one's breath in and out is a popular meditation technique. (There is also walking meditation which incorporates movement.)

A quick Google search can provide you with enough resources and experts on the topic of mindfulness meditation to last a lifetime so there is no need for me to elaborate. But I will tell you this: If the idea of traditional meditation does not appeal to you, you have options.

I am no authority on the subject, but I have invested in reputable meditation programs and given it a try on several occasions. Those experiences taught me enough to know that this route to mindfulness is just not everyone's cup of tea. And it is definitely not the only path.

To tell you the truth, meditation makes me itchy. And sleepy. And often stressed out about how much time it's going to take and whether the kids will get home from school or the phone will ring or I'll get an Amazon delivery while I'm in the midst of it. I find it difficult to fully relax during this style of meditation and I know I am not alone in that.

But, as the Buddhist poet Ikkyu says, "Many paths lead from the foot of the mountain, but at the peak we all gaze at the single bright moon." Yoga, gardening, playing ukulele, and extreme mountain biking can all be paths to mindfulness, too, but they aren't for everyone either.

On the other hand, walking is just so *natural* that it's hard to deny that it *is* for everyone. Whether you're a yogi or a couch potato. So, if you like the idea of getting a little exercise while you practice mindfulness, and you are physically able to walk, even slowly, strolling in the outdoors might just be the path of least resistance for you, as it has been for me.

Why Outdoors?

As you'll see in a later chapter, Nature promotes mindfulness. Not just relaxation and lowered stress, but deep, present moment awareness that you simply cannot get on a treadmill or an indoor track. Beyond that, Nature has significant, measurable effects on the brain and body.

Even if you have never considered yourself a huge

"nature lover", I'd lay odds that, at some point in your life, you've hung a picture on your wall or used a screensaver featuring a natural landscape. Even those of us who spend most of our lives indoors are drawn to images of natural settings. Nature nurtures humans.

Why else do every one of those noise masking apps feature the sounds of wind, rain, ocean waves, birds and crickets? It is part of our DNA to feel better, calmer, stronger and happier when we spend time in Nature and dozens of scientific studies now support the idea. (I'll share some of them in a later chapter.)

Walking is a natural way to move, and spending time in Nature is a natural way to calm our minds, support our bodies, and refresh our souls. Mindful walking is about simultaneously engaging in two healthy activities that we are genetically "pre-programmed" to do and enjoy. And when you find yourself doing something you were meant to do, it feels pretty awesome.

Points to Ponder

- Consider the difference between being "mindful" and being "mindless".
- Can you think of some instances where you have been mindful (intensely focused on the present moment) without even trying? What were you doing?
- What natural settings, images, or elements are particularly appealing to you? How do you feel when you think of them?

4

The Making of a Mindful Walker

At first, walking in my neighborhood was a way to clear my head, relieve some stress, and keep the dog from ruining the new carpet. If I didn't dawdle too much, I figured it could also count as my workout for the day.

Since I had no particular agenda or destination on these walks, it was easy to let my mind wander. When I got tired of running through my laundry list of "problems" or philosophizing in my head, I found myself just sort of... zoning out. I didn't know it at the time, but that's "where the magic happens", as they say. It's the first step toward mindfulness.

It didn't seem to matter whether or not I was actually trying to clear my head; when I took a break and stepped outside for my daily walk, my attention was inevitably eventually drawn to the Nature around me.

I found myself noticing details about the trees, birds, clouds, spider webs, and stones that had never caught my eye before. (Note: I found out later that there is a name for this phenomenon. The natural tendency to be drawn to these kinds of details is called "soft fascination".)

Now, to be honest, I've always considered myself a bit of a "nature girl". I grew up tromping through the woods and rocky fields and forging streams in Western Maryland. When my kids were little, we took them fishing and camping. I still enjoy the occasional mountain hike (in fair weather) and I could walk for miles along the seashore, collecting shells and watching seabirds.

But the "soft fascination" I started to experience on my mindful walks took my experience of the Natural world to a whole new level. The more time I spent outside letting my mind just sort of drift along with my feet, the sharper all my senses seemed to get.

For the first time, I started to feel the texture of gravel under my feet and the way the breeze lifted the hair on my arms. When I looked up (I realize I rarely used to look up), I noticed little things like the shape of a cloud or a squirrel's nest at the very top of a tree. Had that branch always been bent like that? Is that a nest? I pocketed acorns and pinecones and noticed how they prickled against my palms. Sometimes, it felt a little like being a kid again.

Often, while I was doing nothing more than walking and observing, something would shift inside me and I experienced an overwhelming feeling of contentment, as though all was right with the world. I might walk for ten minutes in this state or it might stretch to 30. However long it lasted, while it did, life just seemed manageable. I felt supported, connected, and strong. Every time this happened, I came home feeling better than I had when I left.

Before long, I was hooked on these mindful walks.

For a few minutes each day, I stopped worrying about what would happen next week or reminiscing about my old life. I started to look forward to my regular break from thinking about the unpacked moving boxes or the bills or the business. I really lived in the present, maybe for the first sustained time ever. (Most of us have had moments of intense present-moment awareness, but they're typically fleeting.) Best of all, the more I walked, the better I felt—both mentally and physically.

My weight evened out and started to notice a new firmness in my middle and a nice shape to my calves. (I might sell more copies of this book if I just focused on those things!) But I also found that, when I returned to my home office after even 15 minutes or so of mindful walking, I got more done, felt more energetic and focused, and was more patient with everyone around me.

Within a few weeks of walking daily, problems that might have seemed daunting—or at least caused me a day or so of hand-wringing—a month earlier felt like less of a "big deal". Mindful walking wasn't just calming me down and relieving some stress. It was actually making me more creative and resilient.

A word about Stress

We have all heard the warnings about the negative consequences of living with constant stress—even if that stress is relatively low-level. It turns out that those "fight or flight" hormones that surge through our system when we're anxious were supposed to be reserved for *actual* fighting or fleeing. These days, most of us do neither.

Heart disease, cancer, stomach ulcers, autoimmune disorders, weight gain or loss, sleeplessness, and headaches are just some of the conditions linked to unmanaged stress. At the very least, being stressed out makes it harder to lose weight, maintain healthy relationships, concentrate on our work or our goals, or even get a deep breath.

If you found this book with a search term like "stress

relief", you are not alone. Many new mindful walkers find their way to the practice the same way, either intentionally or by happy accident.

Even if you cannot point to a particular source of anxiety in your life, mindful walking is a great, simple tool for keeping it at bay or for restoring equilibrium quickly. Movement releases physical tension while mindfulness and exposure to Nature build mental resilience. Research suggests that people who walk in the outdoors regularly are not only less likely to feel stressed out in the present, but are also more likely to be able to manage stressful situations in the future.

And because it doesn't take much time, effort, or money, mindful walking is unlikely to *add* to your stress level!

I had worked out for years, but had never experienced such long-lasting and far-reaching effects from my hours of watching "House Hunters" while I walked on the gym treadmill. When I became a mindful outdoor walker, I smiled more, slept better, kept my weight in check (less need for late night stress binging!) and even started to have some new insights about my life. It was almost as though I had stumbled onto a secret super power.

The amazing thing is. . . I had. And so can you.

Points to Ponder

- Can you think of a time when being in the outdoors made you feel better? (Even if you have to think way back) Do you think it still could?
- What are the biggest stressors in your life right now? What are you doing to offset their potentially damaging effects on your body, mind, and spirit?
- Shakespeare said "The earth has music for those who listen." What "music" might you need to hear?

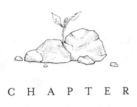

5

Is This the Path for You?

If you are physically healthy enough to walk and be outside and you have a desire to take better care of not just your body but your mind and spirit, too, then mindful walking may be a great fit.

Whether or not you are currently physically active and regardless of whether you've ever dabbled in meditation, you can start a mindful walking practice this afternoon and start seeing and feeling the benefits immediately.

That's not to say that it won't take a little getting used to. There is not much of a learning curve with mindful walking, but it is a new way of engaging with the world—not just a physical activity, but not a straightforward meditation practice either.

Before I adopted mindful walking as my primary form of exercise, I worked out at a gym a few times a week. At the time, I enjoyed "tuning out" with music or an audiobook while I let my body move more or less "mindlessly".

After I relocated and didn't have a gym (or the money to join one), I tried to walk in the same way outside, with my mind on autopilot and my music cranked up. But it did not work very well.

Walking in the outdoors, where there were so many more sights and sounds, was just so much more engaging. The music became a distraction and an irritation. As soon as I took out my earbuds, slowed the pace a little, and relaxed into the groove of my more meditative walking routine, it was as though I could feel my mind and my body saying "Yes!" I felt an urge to pay more attention, not just to the birds and other Nature sounds, but also to my own internal landscape—my breath, my heartbeat, the feel of my body in space, and the sound of my feet. The overall effect was so much more calming.

Surprisingly (to me, at the time), it was also effective. Even at a slower pace, I managed to maintain my weight, firm up my backside, and create some killer calf muscles. That would not surprise any modern exercise physiologist. Research now shows that being mindful during a workout can increase the effectiveness of exercise, decrease the risk for injury, help us feel more positive about our bodies, and increase overall enjoyment.

Just to be clear: If you're addicted to Pure Barre or Pilates or you are one of those people who gets a big rush from jogging to your favorite music—inside or outside—by all means, keep it up! Physical activities of all kinds offer a myriad of benefits. Thankfully, mindful walking can be an easy, balancing complement to all kinds of other routines. The yin to your fitness yang.

If you don't currently exercise regularly, that's fine, too. Walking is one of the easiest, least expensive, and gentlest forms of movement to get you started. Walking is also one of the safest physical activities for people who are new to regular exercise because it is self-adjusting. It is very hard to "overdo it" while walking mindfully. By definition, you are walking at a pace that is comfortable to you, so it is easy to build your stamina as you build a new habit. Walking is a great all-around physical activity you can do for a lifetime. There is no time like the present to start!

If you have practiced meditation or yoga, there are aspects of mindful walking that will definitely feel familiar but others that will be new. For instance, while you may find it easy to be mindful in the quiet atmosphere of a yoga studio, it may be trickier in your neighborhood or in a public park. After all, it isn't safe to be walking around in a daze!

Instead of relying on the beat of a soundtrack or the guidance of an instructor, mindful walking utilizes the naturally instructive power of Nature and the rhythm of your own breath and movement to help center you in the present moment.

One of the things I love most about mindful walking is that it has the ability to meet you exactly where you are. Everyone's journey is a little different and we need different things at different times in our lives. There is no single "right" pace or method for walking mindfully. (Although I will have some tips in a later chapter.) People come to mindfulness in their own way, in their own time. It can't be forced. In the meantime, the calming and energizing benefits of gentle movement and exposure to Nature can help you get from wherever you are now—physically, mentally, or emotionally—to where you want to be.

A Few of the Benefits of Mindful Walking

Increased Energy (Even when you aren't "feeling it") — For the most part, I like to be physically active. But I have to confess that I have never found a pounding workout to be 'just the ticket' when I'm already exhausted. Is that just me? On the other hand, taking a moderate walk, especially if it can be done outdoors, is a proven way to boost both energy and mood. I sometimes find myself more in the mood for a "real" workout afterward!

A Boost in your Mood — Right from the start of my mindful walking journey, taking short walks not only gave me the chance to let off a little steam, but also kept me from unnecessarily (and unfairly) taking out my frustration on the people around me while I let Nature calm me down. Try it and see. If you don't have time to walk, start by just *standing* outside near something green. Especially if this isn't something you do often, you may find the calming effect quite amazing.

Better Decision Making — According to researchers at Stanford, creative thinking can jump by as much as 60 percent while walking. Although I started walking to deal with frustration and anxiety, I soon discovered that a side benefit of walking in a mindful way was a significant increase in my ability to make meaningful connections and solve problems. Often, answers to tricky problems surface naturally after a short head-clearing walk outside. When overthinking stops, creative thinking can start.

Improved Mental Focus — Ever sit staring at a blinking cursor for longer than you'd like to admit, fingers poised to write that email, report, novel, etc.? Yep, time to walk. According to a 2010 study by University of Illinois psychologists, walking at your own pace for 40 minutes, three times a week, "increases performance on cognitive tasks". I'll take some of that!

Can Help Ward Off Depression — Both physical activity and mindfulness have been shown to have positive effects on mental health. Mindful walking lets you do both at once. When I was dealing with a bunch of major life stressors, I instinctively went outside to "get away from everything". Ironically, I found that quiet, contemplative walking gave me the tools I needed to actually *deal* with the things in front of me (rather than avoid them) and put them in perspective, while simultaneously giving me a deeper appreciation for the many good things in my life and the world.

Do You Have to Be "Spiritual" to Be a Mindful Walker?

In a word, no. One beautiful aspect of mindful walking is that anyone can do it and receive the benefits. Although the modern understanding of mindfulness is an adaptation of the Buddhist concept of *Sati*, the secular version is all about awareness.

Molecular biologist Jon Kabat-Zinn is credited with popularizing this secular concept of mindfulness, which he defines as "the awareness that arises through paying attention on purpose in the present moment, and nonjudgmentally." (In this context, nonjudgmentally can be understood to mean "without forming an opinion". In other words, you just don't engage with your thoughts while you walk. You let them go.)

You don't have to be religious, spiritual, or into yoga or meditation to walk mindfully in Nature. Likewise, you can be any size, shape, gender, or age. You can be an outdoorsy person or a bookworm (or an outdoorsy bookworm like me!). Importantly, you also don't have to be able to understand how the components of mindful walking work together in order for them to still work wonders for you.

Although you'll read words like soul, intuition, and "spirit" in this book, the process of mindful walking is actually very down-to-earth and grounded in scientific evidence. (*See Chapter 6*) Exposure to Nature induces measurable changes in heart rate, blood pressure, cortisol (the stress hormone) level, and brain activity. Regular physical activity positively impacts nearly every health metric. It also triggers production of brain-derived neurotrophic factor (BDNF), a protein that has been called "fertilizer for the brain", and lowers disease risk. Mindfulness and meditation trigger an increase in alpha brain waves which can change how we think and behave. Those are facts. And they are pretty exciting.

But some people may still ask, *"Is there a spiritual aspect to mindful walking?"* The answer is, it depends.

On one hand, you may simply want to use mindful walking as a powerful way to release stress, boost energy, improve your health, and become more mentally focused, all of which are reasonable expectations.

On the other hand, many people find that the act of creating some space in their overcrowded lives to mindfully commune with Nature opens a channel into a deeper, more spiritual part of themselves. Personally, I do feel a deep connection with the Divine when I walk, though it is different—and often more personal— from what I experience in church. Connecting with the Natural world reminds me that I am connected to something bigger than myself and, for me, that bigger something is God.

Whether or not you experience any kind of spiritual awakening, evidence suggests that you stand to gain far more from mindful walking than you might expect from a ten to fifteen minute investment.

As someone who has experienced significant physical, emotional, and spiritual benefits from the practice, I encourage you to just stay open. There is nothing you have to do. There is no destination.

Maybe you're already a lifelong walker or a person with a highly-evolved consciousness and you're familiar with the spiritually transforming power of walking in Nature. (If so, enjoy your walks and pass this book along to a friend!)

But if you are more like I was, a curious but open-minded skeptic who can't necessarily define the word "namaste", know that you don't have to understand or even believe in all that a practice like this can do in order to experience the benefits. Just open your door, take that first step, and see where it leads.

Points to Ponder
- What is your favorite physical activity? How might mindful walking complement what you are already doing?
- If you do not currently engage in regular physical activity, could you see yourself taking a few short walks a week? If not, what might stand in your way?
- Do you see mindful walking as a "spiritual" practice? Why or why not?

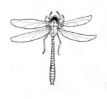

6

The Science Behind Mindful Walking

I didn't invent mindful walking, of course. I wasn't even the first one to discover it.

Some of the greatest philosophers, artists, scientists, and theologians from Socrates to Wordsworth to Einstein have been avid outdoor walkers. Einstein advised "Look deeply into Nature and you will understand everything better." The Naturalist John Muir wrote, "In every walk with nature one receives far more than he seeks." Even Nietzsche observed that "It is only ideas gained from walking that have any worth."

Long before there was any scientific evidence to back them up (and now there is plenty), many creative types seemed to know intuitively that there was something powerful and almost magical about placing our feet on the Earth and moving mindfully through the Natural World. They sensed that attuning to green spaces, bird-song, and fresh air made them calmer, boosted their energy, and helped them focus.

Now, Science is starting to catch up with ancient wisdom. Below is a small sample of some of the most relevant recent findings on walking, mindfulness, and connecting with Nature. If you are curious, I encourage you to do your own Internet search and see what you find. New studies are being released all the time.

- People who live in "walk friendly" neighborhoods, which are defined as neighborhoods where they can walk to grocery stores, schools and shops, have significantly less evidence of high blood pressure, diabetes, and obesity, according to the Institute for Clinical Evaluative Sciences in Toronto

- In a 2014 Stanford University study entitled "Give Your Ideas Some Legs," researchers found that people scored higher on several different creativity tests both during and right after walks.

- According to a study by the Lawrence Berkeley National Laboratory in California, a brisk walk can reduce the risk of heart disease more effectively than running.

- Practicing mindfulness, or present moment awareness, has been shown to reduce the size of the amygdala, the brain's "fight or flight" center and the source of fear and anxiety. You read that right. Mindfulness *can physically alter the brain.*

- A recent study in Scotland found walkers' brains became calmer and more meditative in green spaces than in urban environments.

- A number of studies have found that exposure to phytoncides—compounds released by trees such as pines, cedars and oaks—can lower blood pressure, relieve stress and boost white blood cell count.

- Research published in *Psychological Science* finds that we engage in what researchers call "creative incubation" when we take time to "zone out".

- A 2010 University of Essex study found that even small amounts of outdoor exercise can have remarkable beneficial effects on mental health.

- Being in nature makes people feel more alive, according to a series of studies published in the June 2010 issue of the *Journal of Environmental Psychology.*

And the list goes on and on.

Is it Too Simple?

So, there is good science on the benefits of each of the three components of mindful walking: mindfulness, walking, and communing with Nature. Even before I became really intentional about my mindful walking practice, it was evident that the more I walked, the better I felt and the more I *wanted* to walk. I hadn't yet done a shred of research, but I could already tell that something significant was happening to me.

At the same time, I was spending virtually no money on my new "hobby" and very little time. There was no pain, no pounding, no chanting, no heavy sweating, no special equipment involved, and it made me feel great. Even with minimal time, a new business, and a busy family life, I was managing to take short walks at least a few times a week.

The biggest question for me became, Why isn't everyone doing this?

The answer, of course, is multifaceted. We're busy, we're tired, and we have our routines in place. Economics plays a role, too. We don't all live in "walk friendly" neighborhoods or have easy access to forests, beaches, or parks.

But I think the real reason goes deeper than that.

As humans have moved farther away from the daily need to be in contact with Nature for survival, it's just not something we think about. For many people, the journey from the house or apartment to the car and from the car into work or school is the extent of our "outside time" on most weekdays. Even the weekends are mostly spent indoors.

According to the Environmental Protection Agency, the average American spends 93% of their life indoors. About six percent of that is spent in our cars. My personal theory is that the idea of intentionally spending time doing something as simple as walking in Nature is so simple that it pretty much flies beneath the radar in our more "highly-evolved" lives.

And yet... couldn't your life use a little more simplicity?

Forget the Research
Now that you have seen a little bit of the research on mindfulness, walking, and Nature connection, forget it.

Instead, just listen to your own body. Our bodies are far wiser and more intuitive than we give them credit for. Put your hand on your heart. Close your eyes. Breathe deeply. If you're feeling stiff, sluggish or "out of shape", chances are you know that you need to do something. (It may be what drove you to pick up this book!)

While you're debating your many options, why not start with a short mindful walk? The scientific research, my own experience, and that of countless others a lot smarter than me all support the idea that getting outside for a little mindful walking has the power to not only make us healthier, but also transform the way we live, work, think, and interact with the world.

Do I have your attention yet?

C'mon. . . Let me show you the path!

Points to Ponder

- Why do you think Nature walks have been favored by so many thinkers and creators throughout history?
- Can you remember the last time you intentionally went for a walk outdoors, just for walking's sake? How did it feel?

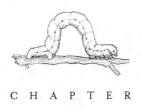

CHAPTER

7

The Three Elements of Mindful Walking

As you may have figured out by now, mindful walking is simply the practice of walking in the outdoors without thinking about much of anything, but rather sensing and feeling our inner and outer worlds instead. It's about as straightforward as that. Although, by practicing some of the techniques I'll teach you, it is possible to optimize the benefits to both your mind and body and get even more "bang for your buck", so to speak.

But I would be remiss if I didn't tell you the truth – that if you stopped reading right now and just went out and walked quietly in Nature for a few minutes every day for the rest of your life, the entire trajectory of your life would very possibly change. Everything, from your work to your relationships to your health and your sleep, would improve and the things that cause you stress right now would gradually fade into the background of the Bigger Picture that is you.

You would discover—because it can't help but well up from inside you if you let it—a unifying source of Wisdom, Strength, Energy, and Bliss that is not only readily available to all of us in every moment but is, in fact, our birthright. This is not an exaggeration.

However, since you are still reading, I am assuming that you could use a little more information and maybe even some practical guidance in how the practice of mindful walking actually works and, more importantly, how to put it to work for you. Not to worry. I've got you covered.

Let's start with the basics.

Three Essential Elements

Mindful walking relies on three elements, each of which is essential to the power and effectiveness of this simple practice. The three elements are Nature, Movement, and Mindfulness (also known as present moment awareness).

Of course, as we've seen in Chapter 6, you can gain many benefits by exposing yourself to any one of these three elements by itself. You can be mindful, *or* exercise, *or* enjoy fresh air and all three can help make you healthier, happier, and more peaceful. But the *real* magic happens when you put them together!

In the next three chapters, we'll break each of them down. Although I refer to these three elements as "Steps" in the chapter titles, keep in mind that they aren't really sequential. When you get outside, get moving, and get present at the same time, it creates a powerful synergy that sets mindful walking apart from other mind/body practices.

The First Step: Get Outside

Remember how great it felt to play in grass when you were a kid? Remember how you couldn't wait to get home from school and run around outside? Remember how freeing and relaxing and just plain *fun* it was? What happened to that?

Well, life happens. As we grow up, a lot of us just end up feeling too busy and time-pressed to "waste" time outdoors, except, maybe, when we're on vacation or enjoying a weekend golf game. Unless you have a job that happens to take you outside, it's entirely possible that the only time you spend in the outdoors during a typical workweek is the time it takes you to walk from your car into a building and back.

Remember that EPA estimate that most of us will spend 93 percent of our lives indoors? (That includes childhood, by the way.) Well, that percentage is growing as more people move away from areas with lots of green spaces into more urban centers.

And yet, study after study (*see Chapter 6*) confirms what you can feel for yourself if you step outside into a green space right now: Nature makes us calmer, improves our mood, boosts our self-esteem, releases stress-busting endorphins, and makes us feel more peaceful.

Ask yourself this question and then quietly listen for the answer that will rise up from inside you. (And while you're at it, say 'hello' to the person giving you that answer. That's your Intuitive Self!)

Was I really born to spend my life indoors, gazing wistfully at inspirational landscape wallpaper on my computer screen?

I don't think so either.

That's why an outdoor setting is a key part of the power in a mindful walking practice. It's the "secret sauce", if you will, that separates this simple practice from other mind-body exercises such as yoga or Tai Chi. Not that these cannot also be practiced outside —they can, and often are. The difference is that mindful walking *depends* on green spaces more than it depends on technique. Nature is central.

You say you don't live in a park? Not a problem! Can you see a tree *somewhere*? Is there grass beside your nearest sidewalk? Can you see the sky? That's all you need.

The idea is simply to be *outside*, in the presence of whatever "nature" happens to be near you. If you have time and are inclined to drive to a park or a bigger green space than whatever is right outside your door, that's fine, too. Just don't feel like you have to go too far. That will just give you another reason not to do it.

One of the key beauties of mindful walking is that it is readily accessible and can be done quickly, almost anywhere. And who knows? Your new mindful walking practice might just prompt you to go find some green spaces in your area that you didn't even know existed. A number of cities have constructed walking trails and greenways designed to accommodate our growing awareness that Nature is central to human wellbeing.

A Word About Setting

Some people get very hung up on the idea that they don't have an "appropriate" place to practice mindful walking and they let it keep them from even getting started. I almost put the word "nature" in the subtitle of this book but took it out at the last minute for fear that it might put off people who don't happen to live in the woods or on a beach.

You don't have to live in a rural or even a suburban

setting to make this work for you. Yes, it is important to walk in the most natural outdoor setting you can find, simply because of all the aforementioned benefits of green spaces. And, yes, it's nice if you can find a relatively quiet place because it is conducive to mindfulness.

But if a city sidewalk with concrete planters or a nearby garden store or greenhouse is what is accessible to you, so be it. If that's the case, really just enjoy the warmth of the sun on your skin as you walk, look up and watch the clouds, try to spot a squirrel or a "volunteer" dandelion in sidewalk cracks. Practice becoming so quiet inside that a butterfly might land on you. Having to become hyper-aware and really *look* for the Nature around you can even help you become more mindful!

Note: *To help you keep experiencing the healing properties of natural elements even after your walks, I have a free downloadable audio training. You can grab it now (before you forget!) at TheMindfulWalker.com/instant-raise*

Points to Ponder

- What is the nearest place where you could take a mindful walk? What do you like or not like about this setting?
- Does your town have trails or greenways you might want to explore?

C H A P T E R

9

The Second Step: Get Moving

There is something about moving our bodies in gentle, rhythmic ways, that allows our brains to relax and "disengage". That is why some people love to dance and others swear by jogging or swimming. As a kid, I could swing on a swing set for hours. When we get into "the zone" in any activity, we are able to temporarily tune out the world and center ourselves in the present, something that has repeatedly been shown to facilitate creativity, planning, and problem solving. (Yes, this is essentially mindfulness but we're not to that chapter yet. See, I told you these all worked together!)

We also now know that movement is essential for our physical health. Exercise that gets our bodies moving and our hearts pumping increases strength and flexibility, releases stress-busting endorphins, lowers the risk for chronic diseases and boosts heart health. Again, if you did nothing more after reading this book than simply start walking regularly, you would enjoy a range of physical and mental benefits.

Of course, we are going to take this a few steps further.

But before we do... consider this: What is the easiest whole-body movement you can think of? One you have been doing since childhood? One that is easy on the joints, requires no technique, no instruction, no particular level of physical fitness or prowess, and won't get you funny looks if you happen to be seen engaging in it outside? You guessed it. (Well, you better have guessed it!) Simple walking.

Add to that the fact that you don't need special equipment, special clothing, a special setting or special *anything* and it's clear why walking is a perfect go-to choice to get moving, especially when time or money is limited.

Beyond that, walking is a method of moving around that we, ourselves, did not invent. How cool is that? People came up with dancing and tennis and Pilates and skiing and mountain biking. All of which can be fun and effective ways of exercising and interacting with the world and our fellow humans.

But walking is effortless, beyond thought, beyond planning. Almost like magic, walking propels us through green spaces at *exactly* the right speed to fully notice and appreciate subtle natural cues at a level that is not possible when we are flying by them in a moving vehicle or even on a bicycle. It's almost as though we were *created* to be walkers.

News Flash: *We were.*

Movement Tips

The best way to start a mindful walking habit is to simply start. Don't think about it too long, don't spend too much time planning, and don't worry about whether or not you will know how to get it right. The first step is to take the first step. Below are some loose "instructions" to help you get started. Understand, though, that your own personal experience of the practice will develop and evolve as you do it. Trust me. It will.

Pace: To get the most out of a mindful walk, start by establishing a steady pace, not so fast that you could not carry on a conversation, but not so slowly that it feels like just "ambling" along. The steady rhythmic sound of your feet making contact with the earth is part of what helps to calm your mind and hone your focus. Get into a groove.

Breath: Practice breathing deeply, filling your lungs so that your abdomen expands with each breath. Exhale completely. As with meditation, mentally "following" the flow of your breath in and out also helps you move naturally into greater present moment awareness. Some people find it helpful to breathe in through the mouth and out through the nose, but there is no set way to do this. As you breathe, remember the Hebrew word for 'spirit', ruah, is synonymous with 'breath'. There is power in purposeful breathing.

Posture: As you move, imagine keeping your chest open. (Note: In some traditions, this part of the body is known as the 'heart chakra', center of love, warmth, compassion and joy. Also, coincidentally, this heart center is associated with the color green!) Your shoulders should be pulled slightly back with your chin in a neutral position and your arms should swing freely. Engage your abdominal muscles gently (too much can hurt your back) and tighten your kegels for an extra punch. This "power stance" sets you up for maximum physical and mental benefit from each step.

Feet and Legs: To engage all of your leg muscles as you walk and get the maximum physical benefit from each step, hit the ground firmly with each heel, rolling your foot all the way through the step, and push off with your toes. With each step, become aware of the solidity and stability of the ground beneath your feet. Imagine it filling you with strength and power from the soles up. If you are moving at a comfortable pace and moving your muscles purposefully and rhythmically, this should feel great!

Points to Ponder

- Do you have some comfortable clothes and supportive shoes that would feel good to walk in? If not, time to shop!
- Have you ever engaged in a physical activity that put you "in the zone"? How did that feel?

C H A P T E R

10

The Third Step: Get Present

Mindfulness has become something of a buzzword in our culture, representing both a practice and a state of mind. Although the practice is rooted in Buddhism, it has also gained a secular following as an effective way to reduce stress and improve overall psychological wellbeing.

I do not pretend to be an expert in mindfulness meditation. In fact, meditation generally makes me sleepy, which is one of the reasons I have come to prefer a more active way of practicing mindfulness through walking.

For the purposes of learning and enjoying mindful walking, the word "mindful" can just be understood to mean "grounded in the present moment". When we walk "mindfully", we are making a real effort to be very aware of and tuned in to what's going on, right this minute, and to temporarily let go of anything that isn't related to that.

By "what's going on", I'm talking about both the external and the internal things that are happening as you walk—a bird flying by, a dog barking, your feet hitting the ground, the smell of the grass, the sensation of your chest rising and falling with each breath. The goal here is not to have a perfectly blank mind, but to calm the static in your brain by focusing only on those things that you can sense in the moment. Engaging as many of your senses as possible is a simple tactic that helps keep your brain too busy for its usual compulsive thinking.

If you've never deliberately tried to do this, it may sound a little crazy that something as simple as just paying attention to the 'here and now' could have such a dramatic impact on our minds and bodies, but the research is compelling.

Among other things, practicing this type of focused awareness regularly has been shown to:

- reduce stress and anxiety
- fight depression
- foster compassion
- improve memory and attention
- boost immunity
- make us feel alive!

Rather than running through your grocery list or planning for your meeting while you take a quick walk around the block, mindful walking invites you to temporarily let go of all of that, breathe deeply, center yourself in the eternal now, and truly *live* the moment in which you are living with all its richness and complexity.

If disturbing or distracting thoughts cross your mind, notice them, acknowledge them, and then let them simply dissipate like mist. This is the nonjudgment we talked about in a previous chapter. If it helps, try actually visualizing that "mist" dissipating out the tips of your fingers or out with your exhaled breath and trailing off behind you as you walk away from it.

When you master this simple exercise, you master your ability to open a mental "door" to a vast source of wisdom, energy, and peace that exists both within and beyond yourself. There are riches to be had in this place.

Mindfulness can take a little practice—especially if you are a planner and a worrier like me—but the results can be nothing short of magical.

Mindfulness Tips

If you are not used to centering yourself in the present moment, don't be discouraged if that stubborn to-do list keeps popping into your head. In fact, if you have the time, there is nothing wrong with using some of your walking time to mull over anything that happens to be on your mind. The outdoors can be a great place to work through problems.

But, when you are ready for true mindful walking —the practice that is going to jumpstart your creativity, improve your sleep, ward off depression, bolster your inner peace, and all that other juicy good stuff—it is important to let all of that go.

How do you do it? *By simply letting go*. Remember, peace is your default setting. Your goal is, therefore, to let your inner stillness surface, rather than try to impose stillness on a busy mind. The quieter you become, the closer you get. Measured breathing, a steady pace, and intentional observation of your natural setting can help. So can some simple visualizations.

When one of those inevitable pesky outside thoughts crosses your mind, simply acknowledge it without engaging with it, and then try to visualize yourself releasing that thought or worry with your exhaled breath.

Above all, don't waste your precious mindful walking time beating yourself up for just doing what we humans do. Thinking (and overthinking) are long-time habits for most of us. Instead of trying to push thoughts out of your consciousness, which often has the opposite effect, simply allow them to breeze right through you and out the other side. Leave them in your wake and remember that whatever is on your mind will still be right there waiting for you when you return from your walk.

But, by then, you're going to be prepared to handle it with more grace and equanimity.

Although mindful walking is pretty easy, it can be a lot to remember when you are getting started and having a guide can be helpful. To help you get started on the right foot (or the left), I've recorded a short audio program that is a perfect companion to this book, which is part of your Book Bonuses. You can download it for free at TheMindfulWalker.com/BookBonuses

This 10-minute guided audio program is designed to do a couple of things. First, it can help you establish a steady, rhythmic pace which is central to "getting in the groove" of a mindful walk. I've also included some instructions to help focus on and guide your breathing for optimal relaxation and invigoration. When you get both the pacing and the breathing right, a state of mindfulness is almost inevitable. To help you stay in that healthy place for the duration of your walk, I've also included some simple guided visualizations designed to help you release anxieties and quiet a busy mind.

And to help you stay on the path to a healthier, happier, more peaceful life, even *after* your walks, be sure to claim the free audio training and PDF guide on bringing natural elements into your home or workspace. You can get it for free at TheMindfulWalker.com/instant-raise.

Points to Ponder

- Consider what "mindfulness" means to you. What are some reasons you are drawn to the concept?
- What habitual thought patterns might stand in the way of being truly mindful as you walk? Do you think you could give them up for a little while?

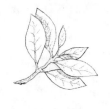

11

Creating Space in Your Life for Mindful Walking

While the beneficial effects of your regular walks will grow the more you walk, there is nothing in particular that you have to do to start this transformation other than put on your shoes and head out the door. There are, however, a few things you need to have in place in order to start off on the "right foot", so to speak.

Mindful walking is the ideal all-in-one mind/body practice for time-pressed people. But the first thing you will need to find (even before you dig out your tennis shoes) to start using its power in your life is *time*. Many people like the fact that mindful walking can tick a lot of important boxes in a short amount of time. Exercise? Check. Self care? Check. Meditation? Check. But you won't be checking any of those imaginary boxes if you can never seem to find the time to get it done.

I know it may seem a little strange to have a chapter on time management in a book about walking mindfully. But I felt it was important to include since "I don't have time" is the *number one objection* I hear from people that keeps them from enjoying all the benefits of this wonderful, healthy practice.

If you have all the time in the world, or if you are incredibly disciplined and are sure you'll never use "busyness" as an excuse to skip a walk, feel free to bypass this chapter.

For the rest of you, I have assembled a few practical tips, based on my own experience as a business owner and mom, that might make it a little easier to find the time you'll need. Implementing even a couple of these tips will improve the odds that, once you start walking, you will have the chance to experience the big payoffs that come from sticking with it.

How Much Time Is This Going to Take?

The good news is that mindful walking doesn't have to take much time at all. Nothing like the amount of time you might devote to, say, a gym workout or a yoga class. I and many others have found that ten to fifteen minutes at a shot is all you need to clear your mind, connect with your intuition, renew your energy, and dramatically raise your feeling of inner peace. Let's find your fifteen minutes!

The first thing we have to acknowledge is that we all have the same 24-hour span in which to get done everything that really matters to us. Finding a few minutes a day (or even every couple of days) for something that could lower your blood pressure, improve your sleep, boost your creativity and problem solving skills, connect you more fully with your higher self, relieve stress, and tone your rear end really comes down to priorities.

If the list above just doesn't excite you, you may not yet be ready for a mindful walking practice. That's fine. We are all at different places on our life journeys and the timing may not be right for you.

On the other hand, if there is something inside you telling you that you really want all of these benefits but you honestly aren't quite sure how you will make it happen given your schedule, hooray! I am about to show you some proven techniques for reclaiming a few minutes of your day, starting now.

Note: *I'm assuming that, if you truly are intrigued by the potential benefits of mindful walking, you're already prepared to cut down on things like binge watching Netflix, browsing Amazon, or checking your social media. So let's start by looking at some other things that are major time leaks for a lot of busy people.*

Batch Your Emails (and other mundane tasks)

According to Fortune magazine, the average adult receives 147 emails a day. Even if your own number falls well below that, it is likely that dealing with digital communications, particularly email, consumes at least a portion of your day.

Although it can be tempting to answer emails as they are received—and it can seem like you're saving time by not leaving them to deal with later—efficiency experts tell us that managing our email in this way is actually inefficient and here's why: Every time your mind is pulled away from the task you were working on, it can take several minutes (up to 23 minutes, actually) to get back to where you were, mentally.

I know, I know. It doesn't seem like it. And it's a drag. But the science doesn't lie. We were not, alas, built for multitasking.

But here's what's great.

You can cut out at least ten minutes (and quite possibly more) *every single day* by limiting email to specific times of the day—say 9, noon, and 3. If you are a compulsive email checker and can't stand this idea, try once every two hours. If you are worried about what people will think, do what Tim Ferris, author of *The Four-Hour Work Week*, suggests and set up an autoresponder letting people know about your policy and giving them an idea when they can expect to hear back from you.

Unsubscribe

On a related note, most of us have signed up to email lists in the heat of the moment and regretted it later. Maybe it was to get a coupon or to access a particular piece of content. And then we just stay on those lists. The emails keep coming after the infatuation has faded and we just don't have the heart or the time to take the 15 seconds needed to get off the list. And that, of course, is what the senders are hoping.

To buy yourself another ten minutes a day of hitting delete in the Promotions tab of your Inbox, take ten minutes today to unsubscribe from the lists that are not really serving who you are now, or who you want to become. Alternatively, you can use a service like Unroll.me to funnel marketing emails you want to keep into a single, easily-read message you can tackle once a day.

Schedule It

Most of us live by our calendars. Whether you use a digital calendar or the old-fashioned paper variety, if you anticipate that you may find it hard to remember to walk, then simply schedule a walk as part of your daily routine, especially for the first month or so while you're establishing the habit. Literally, write it down and assign a time to it. If you're using a digital calendar, set a pop-up reminder.

It sounds like a no-brainer, I know. But I'm telling you this because, if you are anything like me, it can feel self-indulgent or even frivolous to actually put on your calendar something that may appear to others to be a "break time", especially in the middle of your day. Consider this your official permission—no, *instruction*—to do it. You deserve this time, you need this time, and the world needs the person you become when you make a centering and health-giving practice like mindful walking a priority in your life.

Don't leave your mindful walking practice to chance. Put a reminder on your phone and, when it beeps, excuse yourself, step outside, and take your ten minutes to recharge. If you work in an office, this could be the first or the last ten minutes of your lunch break or a small space between meetings. Even just walking around the building, looking at the sky, the trees, or the foundation plantings (seriously!) in the right frame of mind can be incredibly renewing.

(And since you're scheduling it anyway, *tell* someone. This is another form of commitment; we all hate to lose face by not doing what we said we were going to.)

Make it a Transitional Activity

Even those of us who feel like we are constantly on the go have tiny bits of down time when we are shifting focus from one activity to another—say, between eating lunch and starting work again, between the end of work and making dinner, or between making dinner and cleaning up the dishes.

By allowing you to clear your mind, release any built-up tension, and center yourself, mindful walking can actually help make transitions easier and more pleasant and help you be more efficient in the task you're about to start.

Work (or get other things done) in Sprints

I am self-employed and I had just launched a new business when I started my daily walking routine. I definitely did not need the added stress of falling behind in my work or having to scramble at the end of the day because I took "time off" to walk. So I went searching for professional advice on managing my time.

I discovered that many gurus recommend a technique that involves setting a timer and focusing on a single task for a set amount of time, then taking a deliberate and time-limited break. While recommendations vary as to the ideal length of "work" versus "break" time (from as little as 25 minutes' work/10 minute break to as long as 90 minutes' work/30 minute break) experts seem to agree that we accomplish more in focused "sprints" of time. To learn more about the technique and find apps to help you implement it, do an Internet search on the "Pomodoro technique".

One key to making this work for you is that your work time must be free of distractions. I recommend closing unneeded computer tabs and silencing phone notifications for the duration of each sprint.

Make Shoes the Easy Part

A lot of books on walking will tell you how important your shoes are. Some even contain whole chapters on choosing just the right walking shoe. If you need help picking a shoe, I recommend that you get one of these books—or just head to a local athletic shoe store—and let the experts help. Good shoes are critical.

My advice for you in the area of shoes is less scientific but may, in the long run, have an even bigger impact on the success of your mindful walking practice.

Make shoes the easy part. By that I mean, make sure you choose shoes that are easy and fast to put on and keep them close at hand. That may mean by the back door, under your desk, or in the back of your car. If you ever find yourself looking at your walking shoes and thinking "I don't even want to hassle with putting them on", then you need a different pair. (I personally have logged more than 6,500 miles in successive pairs of really supportive flip flops!)

Points to Ponder
- Considering your current schedule, how much time would you be willing/able to devote to mindful walking in a typical week?
- Which of the time management tips in this chapter sound workable to you? Can you think of other ideas to create space in your schedule?

12

Lessons Learned from Mindful Walking

Spending more time in Nature and being more mindful has taught me some things about myself, life, and the world. Here are some of the truths I have come to understand while strolling around my neighborhood and what we can all learn from them.

The world is beautiful.

How long has it been since you really noticed something in Nature? Not just the flowers you planted by the mailbox or the basil in a pot on the deck. When did you last hold an acorn, a pine cone, a leaf, a shell, or a wild flower in your hand? As kids, we did this a lot. Once we're grown, not so much. Honestly, I hope that it has been a while for you because you are in for a wonderful treat. This world is chock full of miracles

(How did that tree come out of that little acorn anyway?) and mindful walking is a great way to tune back in to them.

Feeling a little jaded lately? There is nothing like a walk in Nature to begin to restore some of the childlike wonder we were born with. Look for grass or weeds growing in the cracks of rocks or sidewalks, trees shooting up in open spaces, birds nesting in unlikely places, the pattern dew forms on leaves and spider webs. Take time in these moments to ask yourself how the Universe might be calling you to stretch or grow, too. And don't forget to quietly listen for the answer.

The world is big. Few things are *that* important.

If there is one thing that spending time in the Natural world has taught me, it's that this Earth, and whatever force gave rise to it, is pretty awe-inspiring. Just a moment or two of staring into the night sky, at the ocean, or even at a tree—something many of us rarely take time to do—can induce feelings of expansiveness like almost nothing else. We are individuals, yes, but we are also a part of something a whole lot bigger than ourselves. Reflecting on our own place within the great scheme of things can be a little daunting but it can also be freeing, and can give us a better perspective on our personal problems.

The Universe "has your back".

I didn't plant most of the trees I walk by on my daily loop of the neighborhood. And neither did anyone else. This forest sprung up, and is continually nurtured and renewed, by forces beyond my power or comprehension. The Christian Bible reminds us that the "lilies of the field" do nothing to ensure their own welfare, and yet, thanks to the Divine design, they do just fine. How much more-so is this true of us? Feel how stable the ground is under your feet as you walk. We are supported by this Earth and by this Universe, ultimately safe, regardless of our circumstances, in the fold of a higher intelligence.

We are connected to something really big. . . and cool.

No one taught me how to walk, and yet I can do it pretty much perfectly. My hips swing forward and my feet make contact with the ground. My heart beats, my lungs fill and empty. All of this happens with little or no effort on my part. I have that in common with the trees I pass, without whose life-giving oxygen I wouldn't be walking in the first place. And both the trees and I—and the carpenter bees that are making holes in my mailbox post—depend on the sun's energy and the regular rainfall. In other words, we really are in this together, all of us. And we are more dependent on the Natural world than we sometimes realize. I'm convinced that if more of us understood this at a soul level (as mindful walking can help us do), we all might be moved to preserve and protect the Earth a little better than we do.

Resistance is futile (and painful)

Some days, things just "flow" and other days, everything seems hard. Why is that? Mindful walking has taught me that, more often than not, when something feels "hard", it's because it's not what I'm supposed to be doing at that moment, regardless of what my intellect tells me. So I stop resisting and do something else (like take a walk, make a phone call, or even take a nap!). We tend to think we know best about everything, especially as it pertains to us. But what if there was a greater intelligence that knew better? And what if tuning in to that intelligence, by quieting our minds and accessing our intuition, could keep us in "flow" and in alignment with an easier way of doing things, more of the time? Most of Nature exists in a state of effortless bliss. It begs the question, "How does it do that?"

Sometimes you have to go outside to go deeper inside.

Spending time moving in Nature invites introspection. But not in a brooding, woe-is-me sort of way. As we've talked about, green spaces have been shown to actually boost mood, not drag us down. When I spend time walking outside, I often get all sorts of insights about myself and my life that hours of fret and effort at my desk never seem to give me. When I really want to understand some aspect of myself better, I start by taking a mindful walk.

Deprivation and pain are not required to feel healthier and energized.

Mindful walking is not a weight loss plan. It is a life improvement plan. True, you can certainly lose weight by burning extra calories with a regular walking program. But, much more importantly, mindful walking allows you to connect with a deeper, less self-obsessed part of yourself that knows you're going to be just fine, even if you never lose that extra 10 pounds. When you breathe fresh air, move at your own pace, and allow your busy mind to become still and calm, this truth becomes something you know in your bones. And voila! You feel healthier and more energetic and your weight (or any other physical "flaw") ceases to matter so much.

Points to Ponder
- What aspect of mindful walking is most appealing to you? Why?
- What truths might Nature and a more mindful approach to life reveal to you? Are you excited to find out?

13

Mindful Walking in the Real World

If you have made it this far in the book, I feel like I know you well enough to make a few assumptions.

You are probably a seeker like me, and you are serious about finding some new ways of connecting more deeply with yourself and your world. I'm betting that, in a lot of ways, we're kindred spirits. So I feel comfortable enough to make the following confession: I almost didn't write this book. To be honest, I was worried that the concept of mindful walking was just too simple to be taken seriously.

Then again, as a friend of mine pointed out, toilet tissue dispensers and chip clips probably seemed obvious to the folks who invented them. Now, they're indispensable to the rest of us.

I am just a regular busy woman who stumbled into mindful walking and got so excited by my own results that I felt compelled to 1) validate that the benefits I was experiencing weren't imaginary and 2) tell everyone.

So consider yourself told. I've done my part. The rest is in your hands (and feet!). Nothing you have read here will have any impact on your physical, mental or spiritual wellbeing at all until or unless you get up, slip on those walking shoes, and get out there.

With that in mind, I'm wrapping things up with a look at how I have integrated mindful walking into my own life. Your own practice will look different, of course, but I want to give you a vision of what is possible.

My Walking Practice

Not every walk I take is a mindful walk. Sometimes, I still just want to listen to 80s tunes and work up a sweat. Sometimes, I'm keen to spend time with a new audiobook. Sometimes, I like to walk with my neighbor and chat. And sometimes, I really do want to mull over a problem. All of these ways of spending walking time are legitimate and valuable.

But, no matter how many other kinds of walks I take in the course of a week, I know that my mindful walks are central to my wellbeing so I continue to carve out a little time for one, most days. It's not uncommon for me to just breeze up the lane and back with one or more of my dogs, early in the morning, just before I start work.

Because my work schedule is flexible and my office is in my house, I often use a little of my lunch time for a mindful walk. This may or may not be feasible for you, depending on your situation, but I can tell you that, on days when I'm able to take even a 10-minute mindful walk in the middle of the day, I find that I'm less likely to experience that mid-afternoon "slump" that too often sends me running for the nearest Starbucks.

On days when neither of those options is feasible, I will often take a little time for a mindful walk right after supper. (This has the added benefit of ensuring that someone *else* has to pitch in with the kitchen clean-up!) If they are not already on my feet, those flip flops I mentioned (or clogs in the cooler months) stay right by the back door. I also keep a bottle of sunscreen and a hat nearby, because that's the way I roll.

For the first five minutes or so, I typically do nothing more than listen to the birds and my own footsteps, become aware of my breathing, and allow thoughts to drift right through my mind. I like to envision intrusive thoughts and worries dissipating like steam and trailing out from the ends of my fingertips behind me as I walk.

After a few minutes, I direct my awareness to the feel of my body in space. I may roll my shoulders forward and back (most of us carry tension here, so it's a good habit to get into), tilt my head from side to side, and shake out my arms and hands. As we discussed in Chapter 12, I give attention to my feet as they strike the ground, enjoying the comforting solidity of the ground and rolling fully through each step for maximum benefit to my legs and bum. Because it has become a habit now, I usually also keep my abdominal muscles engaged (though never painfully tight) as I move. As with all aspects of this practice, this is optional.

Then... I just... kind of... *be*, and see what happens.

I see and hear and smell things, but I rarely think about them. Instead, I allow myself to *experience* them. I try to give myself the gift of just coexisting in harmony with the Natural world as I move. In this way, I have nearly stumbled over wild deer and squirrels and even, one time, a bear, which barely glanced up as I passed. (I have come to believe, based on my own experience and that of other mindful walkers, that human beings moving through the Natural world in an intentionally mindful way, emit a sort of peaceful "vibe" that just does not seem threatening to other creatures.)

The point is, don't overthink it. Really, don't "think" about it at all. Our habit of constant thinking *can* be overcome and it's soooo worth it. You don't have to give up your precious intellect for good. We're talking about ten to fifteen minutes of your day that will actually *sharpen* your ability to think effectively and creatively afterward.

Follow the time management tips in Chapter 12 to slip in a quick walk when the opportunity presents itself, even if it's just a couple of times a week, and you'll still be doing better—in terms of both movement and mindfulness—than the bulk of the population!

If this concept sounds intriguing or inviting to you, it probably means there is a part of you that knows you need this in your life. I believe you should honor that and I really want to support you in making it happen.

Mindful walking launched me on a journey of discovery on which I continue to travel daily. This book is my invitation to you to join me on this path. Imagine how the world might be different if more of us were mindful walkers!

If you like what you've heard here and could use some ongoing encouragement and support to help keep you in mindful connection with the Earth, please visit me at TheMindfulWalker.com. There are many free resources there and I regularly share new ones. I would be honored to be your guide!

Until we meet again, blessings on your journey and Happy Trails!

14

Ten Mindful Walks

Sometimes, we all need a little help to get started with a new habit. The following pages feature walking prompts excerpted from the card deck, *The Simple Path: 52 Mindful Walks for a Strong Body, a Clear Mind, and a Joyful Spirit.* The deck includes 52 original line drawings from Nature (you have seen a few of them in this book) and bite-sized bits of inspiration to get you up and moving, any time of year, in any kind of weather, no matter what kind of day you're having!

I have included some space under each walk for your own notes, thoughts, and observations. (If you enjoy journaling about your walks, look for *Today on My Walk: A Mindful Walker's Journal.*)

Both the card deck and journal are designed to be perfect companions to this book for those committed to being consistent with their mindful walking practice. Learn more about them at The MindfulWalker.com.

∾ One ∾

Think Small

Feeling unmotivated but know you need a walk?
When it's hard to get going, think really small.
Commit to a "micro-walk" of two to five minutes
(or even shorter if that still feels too long).
Setting a very tiny goal can often overcome the
brain's resistance and a five-minute walk may
effortlessly turn into eight or ten.

If it doesn't, you still win! Acknowledge and
release your lack of motivation, celebrate
achieving your tiny goal, and rest in a quiet
outdoor spot for a few minutes to "recharge".

Breathe Into Presence

Breath work is a proven way to quiet the mind and
open our hearts to messages in the Natural world.
Try this time-honored deep breathing exercise:
As you walk at a comfortable pace, inhale to the
count of four steps, hold for four steps, exhale for
four steps, and pause your breathing for four steps.
Repeat as many times as you like while you walk.
Relax your shoulders downward on each exhale
and practice releasing the worries of the day as
you feel the "dust" of your mind settle.
Smile on the inside.

∽ *Three* ∽

Walking in Circles

Your mindful walks don't always have
to happen on a visible path.
Today, try walking a 'circle of protection'
or a 'circle of love' around your home.
Exit through your front door and walk with
your heart closest to your dwelling.
Whether you're a homeowner, an apartment
dweller, or you live in a yurt, walking the ground
around it is a way to honor and show gratitude
for your sacred space on the Earth.

....

....

....

....

....

....

....

....

∽ Four ∽

A Gratitude Walk

When we become truly mindful of our place in the
Natural World, we begin to see how all things form
a web for our support and enjoyment.
Be conscious of this as you walk today, offering
a moment of gratitude for each "gift" as you notice
it. Give thanks to trees for oxygen and wood, for
cooling and protecting our outdoor spaces,
and for keeping the soil in place.
Send love to the sun for warmth, energy, and light.
Thank the birds for their mood-lifting songs.
Extend vibrations of gratitude through the
soles of your feet for the solidity of the ground
or the softness of the grass.
See how everywhere you look,
the Earth gives us things to be grateful for!

∾ *Five* ∾

Seeing Deeply

We often look at Nature but rarely see it deeply.
Let's change that!
Pause on your walk today to observe a natural
item like a tree, puddle, acorn, leaf, or stone.
Without taking your eyes off the item, try
to make a mental list of 10 to 25 words
to describe how it looks.
Don't give up early!
You are training your brain to look beyond
the obvious. Incorporate this exercise into your
walks from time to time and watch your
powers of observation improve.
Seeing is understanding is appreciating.

....

....

....

....

....

....

....

∽ Six ∽

Jumpstarting Creativity

Need some fresh ideas? Creativity and
problem-solving skills soar when we
spend time in Natural places.
Research shows that a 25 minute mindful walk
in any green space is enough to relax the brain
and trigger flashes of insight. (As an added bonus,
the blue of the sky also enhances creativity.)
To jumpstart your idea generator, stretch your
arms and neck well (most of us carry tension
here), then walk steadily, looking upward
as often as possible.
Imagine your mind as an open vessel into
which the Universe can pour all sorts of
creative solutions!

Mindful "power walking"

What do you think of when you hear the term "power walking"? Maybe speed walkers with gyrating hips?

While it is perfectly possible to be mindful at a speed-walking pace (although you might miss some of the scenery!), mindful "power walking" has nothing to do with speed.

To start, adopt a power stance: Raise your chin, move your shoulders down and back, gently tighten your core, and feel your deep connection to the Earth extending down through your feet. Imagine energy travelling from the Earth's center, up your legs and into your own core with each step. You are a powerhouse!

∽ Eight ∽

Off the Beaten Path

Don't live in a forest but love the idea of
"forest bathing"?
Research shows we can get all the benefits
of forest bathing in just about any outdoor
space when we are mindful.
Today, you're encouraged to walk
in an unfamiliar (safe) location.
If you normally walk in town, head for
a park, greenway, or forest path.
If you normally walk in the woods, seek out
an urban park or outdoor shopping mall.
New places sharpen our senses, ward off
boredom, and invite us to be fully present
(i.e., mindful). Practice non-judgment (lack
of opinion) as you observe some new
sights, scents, and sounds.

....

....

....

....

....

....

∾ *Nine* ∾

Singing in the Rain

Are you a fair-weather walker?
You may be missing out!
Rain-drenched sidewalks, dripping trees, and
damp grass have a beauty—and even an earthy
smell called petrichor—all their own.
As you stroll, consider that water makes up
71 percent of the planet and up to 60 percent
of your own body and is recycled infinitely.
If you're alone, take advantage of the solitude
to splash through a puddle or catch raindrops on
your tongue. Feel your deep connection to Nature
through the water that sustains all living things.

∽ Ten ∽

Active Listening

Shhhh. Did you hear that?
If you're like most people, probably not.
We spend more time tuning out extraneous
noises than tuning in to them.
Mindful walking invites you to do the opposite.
On today's walk, see how many sounds you
can identify, starting with the sound of your own
feet. Notice how you hear just a handful at first
(a bird, a lawnmower, a dog), but it becomes
easier to hear more things the more you walk.
That's Nature's magic "waking up" your sense
of hearing and deepening your connection to
your surroundings.

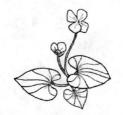

*Take your walking journey
a step further. . .*

I hope that you have enjoyed this book. But, even more importantly, I hope that you have enjoyed experimenting with a deeper, more consistent connection with the Natural World. This book is meant to be an introduction to the practice of communing mindfully with Nature. If you are inspired to take this concept further, integrating more of the Earth's wisdom into your life and work, the following resources may help. Some are things I have created and others are resources that have helped me along my own path.

A downloadable walking meditation and five-day mini-course in mindful walking:

TheMindfulWalker.com/five-day-course

An audio guide and PDF featuring fun ways to boost your energy, focus, and productivity by bringing some Nature inside:

TheMindfulWalker.com/instant-raise

Creative green practices to connect with the Earth in your daily life:

Living Earth Devotional by Clea Canaan
(Note: I read this one daily)

My favorite book of prayers and meditations for honoring the Earth:

Earth Prayers from Around the World
by Elizabeth Roberts and Elias Amidon

Research-based books on how being outside can transform our brains and our lives:

The Nature Fix: Why Nature Makes Us Happier, Healthier and More Creative by Florence Williams

The Nature Principle: Reconnecting with Life in a Virtual Age by Richard Louv

A simple explanation of walking meditation:

The Long Road Turns to Joy by Thich Naht Hahn

A thought-provoking book on plant-human communication:

Thus Spoke the Plant by Monica Gagliano

A wonderful exploration of the power of trees and the role they play in our lives:

The Songs of Trees: Stories from Nature's Great Connectors by David George Haskell

Seven lovely walks to help you experience the benefits of being mindful in Nature:

Natural Mindfulness: Your personal guide to the healing power of Nature Connection by Ian Banyard

Groups devoted to promoting appreciation for and restoration of the Earth:

Treesisters.org
Healingforest.org

Two books about getting clear on what really matters and making time for it:

Essentialism: The Disciplined Pursuit of Less by Greg McKeown

Clarity: Clear Mind, Better Performance, Bigger Results by Jamie Smart

For ongoing encouragement, practical resources, and a tribe of women on a similar path:

TheMindfulWalker.com/collective

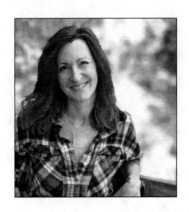

About the Author

Alex Strauss is a writer, coach, and certified Natural Mindfulness guide whose work is accredited by the International Mindfulness and Meditation Alliance. She is a graduate of Wake Forest University and holds an MA in Journalism from American University. Alex lives on the edge of a forest in the beautiful Piedmont region of North Carolina with a handful of her favorite people, dogs, cats, reptiles, and fish. She is a proud member of most North Carolina museums, makes amazing marshmallows, plays the Celtic drum, and still uses her library card.

To connect with Alex and find out more about working with her, visit AlexStraussOnline.com.

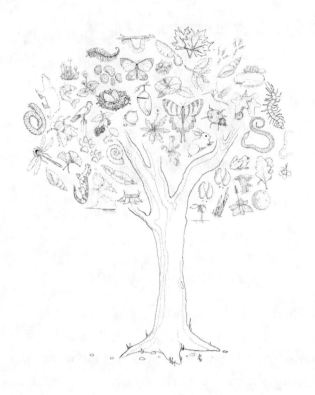

About the Artwork

Each illustration in this book was hand-drawn digitally using a Huion© drawing tablet and Sketchbook© drawing program. Each drawing was individually created to celebrate both the large and small aspects of Nature. Artist Annika Preheim draws inspiration from her study of zoology and her lifelong love for the natural world.

Acknowledgements

My deepest appreciation goes to the growing community of mindful walkers, Nature lovers, and spiritual seekers whose enthusiasm and love for the Earth inspired me to embark on this journey and to write this book.

The members of my book launch team in particular, for both the First and Second Editions, deserve medals for their feedback, suggestions, and careful proofreading to make sure this book was the best it could be. (Especially in light of the fact that I apparently can't spell the word "meditation" to save my life.)

Finally, I owe a debt of gratitude to my designer and friend Angela Corbo Gier, whose artistry and meticulous attention to detail made this book not only more beautiful, but even more impactful, than it otherwise would have been.